CHAIR YOGA FOR SENIORS OVER 60

A Step by Step Exercise Guide to loosing belly fat, revitalize body systems, Enhanced Mobility for a Flexible and Active Life

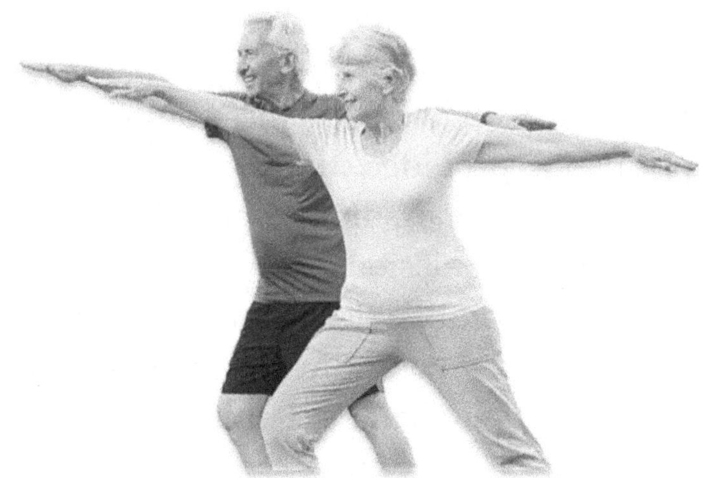

Tracy Parker

The information provided in **"Chair Yoga for Seniors over 60:** *A Step by Step Guide to loosing belly fat, revitalize body systems, Enhanced Mobility for a Flexible and Active Life* " is intended for general informational purposes only. The content within this book is not a substitute for professional medical advice, diagnosis, or treatment. It is crucial to consult with a qualified healthcare professional before beginning any new exercise or wellness program, especially for individuals with existing health conditions, concerns.

While every effort has been made to ensure the accuracy and completeness of the information provided, the author and publisher do not assume responsibility for any errors or omissions. The author and publisher are not liable for any loss or damage incurred directly or indirectly from the use of the information contained in this book.

Readers are encouraged to take personal responsibility for their health and well-being, and any decisions made based on the information provided in this book are at their own risk. The exercises and practices outlined in this book should be approached with mindfulness, and individuals should listen to their bodies, making modifications as needed to ensure their safety and comfort.

By reading **"Chair Yoga for Seniors over 60:** *A Step by Step Guide to loosing belly fat, revitalize body systems, Enhanced Mobility for a Flexible and Active Life,"* readers acknowledge and agree to the terms of this disclaimer. Always prioritize your health and consult with a healthcare professional to determine the most suitable approach for your unique circumstances.

ABOUT THE AUTHOR

Meet Tracy Parker's, the passionate mind behind "**Chair Yoga for Seniors over 60:** *A Step by Step Guide to loosing belly fat, revitalize body systems, Enhanced Mobility for a Flexible and Active Life* ''. With a deep commitment to holistic well-being and a wealth of experience in the field of yoga, Parker brings a unique blend of expertise and empathy to the pages of this transformative guide.

Tracy Parker is a certified yoga instructor specializing in chair yoga, making the practice accessible to individuals of all ages and abilities. Their journey in the world of yoga began with a personal quest for balance and vitality, leading to a profound understanding of the power of gentle movements and mindfulness.

Tracy Parker is known for their compassionate teaching style, guiding students through practices that honor and celebrate the unique capabilities of each individual. Through workshops, classes, and now this comprehensive guide, they share their knowledge, offering a pathway to improved mobility, increased flexibility, and a more vibrant life.

TABLE OF CONTENTS

CHAPTER ONE
Introduction to Yoga

Yoga is a comprehensive system of *mental, physical, and spiritual exercises* that have its roots in ancient India. The Sanskrit root "yuj," which meaning to yoke or connect, is where the term "yoga" originates. Yoga seeks to create a sense of balance and harmony within a person by bringing the body, mind, and soul together.

1. **Physical Aspect**:

-Postures, or Asanas: Yoga consists of a set of physical postures or poses meant to increase balance, strength, and flexibility. Often, these positions are paired with deliberate breathing exercises.

2. **Mental Aspect**: - Pranayama (Breath Control): The technique of pranayama, which entails conscious breath control, is fundamental to yoga. Breathing exercises improve attention and mental clarity by calming and regulating the mind.

- *Dharana (Concentration)*: Yoga uses mindfulness-enhancing and mind-quieting techniques to support the development of concentration. To enter a meditative state, one must be able to focus.

- *Dhyana (Meditation):* A keystone of yoga, meditation entails developing a heightened state of awareness and mindfulness. People aim to achieve a profound sense of inner serenity and unity via meditation.

3. **Spiritual Aspect**: - Yogic philosophy is based on the Yamas and Niyamas, which are moral and ethical precepts. The Niyamas are personal observances like self-discipline (tapas) and contentment (santosha), whereas the Yamas are principles like non-violence (ahimsa) and truthfulness (satya).

-*Samadhi (oneness):* Often referred to be a state of profound spiritual realization and oneness with the divine, samadhi is the ultimate goal of yoga. Reaching samadhi signifies the end of the yogic path.

4. **Yoga Paths:** Bhakti Yoga is the path of devotion, focusing on love and adoration for a supreme being.

- *Jnana Yoga:* The knowledge path that emphasizes discernment, introspection, and the search for the truth.

 Karma Yoga: The path of selfless action, which emphasizes carrying out one's responsibilities without regard to the outcome.

- *Raja Yoga*: A route to spiritual enlightenment through meditation that combines asanas, pranayama, and other techniques.

Yoga is a complete lifestyle that supports well-being on many levels, not simply physical fitness. It is a durable and flexible tradition with broad appeal across the globe because it is an inclusive practice that can be tailored to people of diverse ages, abilities, and spiritual beliefs.

The Multifaceted Benefits of Yoga: Enhancing Physical, Mental, and Spiritual Well-being

Yoga is an age-old discipline with Indian roots that has become well-known for its all-encompassing approach to health and wellbeing. Yoga has several advantages that go well beyond the physical poses, or asanas, that are usually connected with the practice. Yoga, which embraces the mind, body, and spirit, has several benefits that support general health and vigor.

1. Health and Fitness

- Increased number of Motion and Flexibility: Yoga incorporates a number of postures that lengthen and gently stretch muscles, increasing range of motion and flexibility. This improved flexibility lowers the chance of injury and helps with posture.

-Strengthening: A lot of yoga positions call for the activation of different muscle groups,

which enhances general strength and stamina. In contrast to conventional strength training, yoga uses regulated movements and bodyweight resistance to increase strength.

- *Better Balance and Coordination:* Yoga's balancing positions promote stability, which enhances balance and coordination. A major element of this advantage is improved proprioception, or the body's knowledge of its spatial orientation.

- *Joint Health*: Yoga's mild motions lubricate joints, which helps to maintain joint health and may lessen pain brought on by illnesses like arthritis.

- *Cardiovascular Health:* Vigorous yoga styles like Vinyasa or Power Yoga increase heart rate and strengthen the heart. Frequent exercise can support better heart health and circulation.

- *Detoxification:* Yoga incorporates mindful breathing, which activates the lymphatic system and helps the body rid itself of pollutants. In particular, twisting positions are thought to help in detoxification.

2. **Emotional and Mental Health:**

- *Tension Reduction*: Yoga's capacity to lower tension is among its most well-known advantages. Yoga lowers cortisol levels and stimulates the relaxation response in the body through awareness, controlled breathing, and meditation.

- *Reduction of Anxiety and Depression Symptoms:* Regular yoga practice has been linked to a decrease in anxiety and depression symptoms. Mental health benefits from the integration of breathing awareness, meditation, and physical exercise.

- *Improved Sleep Quality:* Yoga helps people unwind and cope with stress, which enhances the quality of their sleep. For those who suffer from insomnia or other sleep disorders, specific poses and relaxation methods might be especially helpful.

- *Mindfulness and Presence:* Yoga's emphasis on breath and body awareness fosters mindfulness, which is the discipline of living in the present moment to the fullest. This increased mindfulness has a positive impact on day-to-day living by encouraging a more composed and balanced response to obstacles.

- *Better Cognitive Function*: Research has connected yoga to improved cognitive function, which includes improved processing speed, memory, and attention. Cognitive health is enhanced by both mental concentration and physical activity.

3. **Spiritual and Holistic Well-Being:** - Spiritual Connection: Although yoga is not intrinsically linked to any one religion, it does offer a means for people to delve deeper into their spiritual lives. The exercise promotes introspection and inner tranquility.

- *Integration of Mind, Body, and Spirit:* Yoga is frequently referred to as a path toward self-realization. By encouraging people to investigate the connections between the mind, body, and spirit, it promotes a sense of completeness and togetherness.

- *Cultivation of Compassion:* The Yamas and Niyamas, or ethical precepts of yoga, encompass virtues like contentment (santosha) and non-violence (ahimsa). Adhering to these guidelines promotes a kind and peaceful attitude toward oneself and other people.

-Stress Resilience: Consistent yoga practice fosters a calm, balanced mindset, which increases resistance to stress. People acquire coping skills that make it easier for them to deal with the difficulties of life.

- Enhanced Energy Flow: The body's life force is known as prana in yogic philosophy. Yoga is said to improve the flow of prana by breath control and particular postures, which results in more energy and a feeling of well-being.

4. **Social and group Advantages:** - Community Connection: Taking a yoga class or becoming a part of a group gives you a sense of connection and belonging. By creating a supportive atmosphere, shared practice motivates people to stick with their well-being journey.

- Mindful Relationships: The tenets of yoga apply to interactions with others in addition to individual practice. Emphasizing understanding, empathy, and compassion

leads to more thoughtful and satisfying interactions.

- Promotion of Holistic Health: People who benefit from yoga's holistic qualities frequently end up advocating for this kind of care. Communities may benefit from this, which would enhance general well-being.

In conclusion, yoga offers a wide range of diverse and extensive health benefits. The practice offers a transforming journey that involves the mind, body, and spirit, going beyond just physical exercise. People of all ages and capacities can discover significant and long-lasting advantages from yoga practice, whether they are looking for physical health, stress relief, mental clarity, or spiritual growth. Yoga is an age-old practice that has endured the test of time, inspiring millions of people worldwide to lead better, more balanced lives.

"Yoga teaches us to cure what need not be endured and endure what cannot be cured." - B.K.S. Iyengar

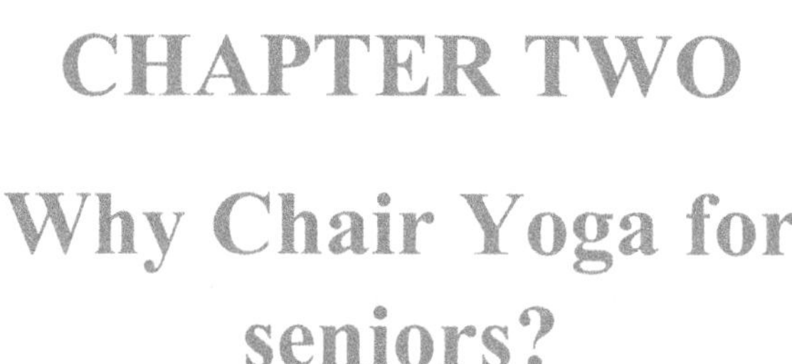

CHAPTER TWO

Why Chair Yoga for seniors?

A modified version of traditional yoga, chair yoga for seniors is designed to meet the demands and physical constraints of senior citizens, especially those who may have mobility, balance, or joint problems. Seniors will find this mild and accessible practice excellent since it may be done while seated or with assistance from a chair. Seniors can benefit greatly from chair yoga, which addresses their physical, mental, and emotional well-being in a comfortable and safe way.

1. **Accessibility and Inclusivity**: A wide spectrum of people, including those with mobility impairments, arthritis, or other physical disabilities, can practice yoga thanks to chair yoga. Seniors can participate comfortably from a chair if they have difficulty getting up and down from the floor or holding certain yoga poses.

2. **Increased Range of Motion and Flexibility**: Chair yoga uses soft stretches and motions that increase range of motion and flexibility without straining muscles or joints. Seniors

who practice regularly can prevent stiffness and promote greater general mobility by maintaining and expanding their range of motion.

3. **Improved Strength and Balance:** Seniors can strengthen their arms, legs, and core by doing standing and sitting poses in this practice. Furthermore, chair-adapted balance poses offer seniors a secure means of improving their stability and lowering their chance of falling, which is a prevalent worry among the elderly population.

4. **Joint Health and Pain Management:** Because chair yoga is mild on the joints, people with arthritis or other joint-related conditions can benefit from it. In addition to promoting joint health, the deliberate motions and emphasis on correct alignment may help relieve chronic pain.

5. **Mindful Breathing and Stress Reduction**: Chair yoga contains regulated breathing techniques and breath awareness, which can help to soothe the nervous system. Seniors can enhance their general mental health, manage

stress, and lessen anxiety by learning and using breathing exercises.

6. **Cognitive advantages**: Mindfulness and meditation, which have been connected to cognitive advantages, are frequently incorporated into chair yoga. Regular chair yoga practice can have a good impact on seniors' focus, memory, and mental clarity, among other benefits.

7. **Social Interaction and Community development**: Seniors can engage in social interaction and community development by taking chair yoga courses. The communal yoga practice in a caring setting can help fight feelings of loneliness and promote a sense of togetherness.

8. **Flexibility to Meet Specific requirements:** Chair yoga is very adaptable to each person's unique requirements and capabilities. Seniors can practice safely and pleasantly since instructors can adjust poses and sequences to suit varying degrees of mobility and fitness.

9. **Promotion of Relaxation and Better Sleep:** Chair yoga incorporates relaxation techniques like mindful breathing and guided

visualization that can help promote better sleep. Chair yoga is frequently discovered by seniors as a means of relaxation and greater rest and recuperation.

10. **Independence and Empowerment:** Chair yoga encourages elders to actively participate in preserving their health and wellbeing. It promotes independence and self-care by offering a mild and approachable type of exercise.

Chair yoga for seniors has many advantages that address the particular requirements of the aging population. Chair yoga offers seniors a fun and safe way to be connected, active, and involved in their wellness journey — from physical fitness and flexibility to mental and emotional well-being. It is a useful and enriching activity for senior citizens looking to improve their general quality of life because of its versatility and inclusion.

How to Overcome Common Misconceptions

Overcoming common misconceptions about chair yoga for seniors involves education, communication, and experience. Here are some strategies to address and dispel misunderstandings:

1. **Educate on the Benefits:**

Provide clear and comprehensive information on the benefits of chair yoga for seniors. Emphasize how it promotes flexibility, strength, balance, and overall well-being. Highlight the adaptability of chair yoga, making it accessible to a wide range of abilities.

2. **Clarify the Purpose**:

Clearly communicate that chair yoga is not a lesser form of yoga but a modified and inclusive approach. Emphasize that it is designed to meet the specific needs of seniors, promoting health and wellness in a safe and comfortable manner.

3. **Show Diversity in Practice:**

Share images and stories that showcase the diversity of individuals participating in chair yoga. This can include seniors of different ages, abilities, and backgrounds. Illustrating the inclusivity of chair yoga can help dispel the misconception that it is only for those with severe limitations.

4. **Address Safety Concerns:**

One common misconception is that chair yoga is not physically challenging. Emphasize that chair yoga can be adapted to varying fitness levels and that it provides a safe environment for seniors to practice. Discuss the importance of proper alignment and how instructors can modify poses to ensure safety.

5. **Provide Testimonials:**

Collect testimonials from seniors who have benefited from chair yoga. Personal stories can be powerful in conveying the positive impact of the practice on physical health, mental well-being, and overall quality of life.

6. Offer Demonstrations:

Conduct chair yoga demonstrations to showcase the variety of poses and exercises involved. Use these demonstrations to highlight that chair yoga is a legitimate and effective form of exercise, dispelling the notion that it is merely a seated, passive activity.

7. Emphasize Mind-Body Connection:

Counter the misconception that chair yoga is solely about physical exercise by emphasizing its holistic nature. Discuss how chair yoga incorporates mindfulness, breathing techniques, and meditation, contributing to mental and emotional well-being.

8. Address Stigma:

Some individuals may resist chair yoga due to perceived stigma associated with age or physical limitations. Foster a positive and encouraging atmosphere by promoting the idea that everyone can benefit from chair yoga, regardless of age or fitness level.

9. Offer Trial Sessions:

Provide opportunities for individuals to experience chair yoga firsthand through trial sessions or workshops. Direct experience can be a powerful way to dispel misconceptions and showcase the practicality and effectiveness of chair yoga.

10. Engage with the Community:

Engage with the senior community through informational sessions, workshops, or outreach programs. This direct interaction allows you to address concerns, answer questions, and build trust among seniors who may be skeptical about trying chair yoga.

11. Encourage Open Communication:

Create an open and inclusive space where seniors feel comfortable expressing their concerns or misconceptions. Encourage dialogue and address individual fears or reservations about chair yoga in a supportive manner.

By combining education, demonstration, and community engagement, you can gradually overcome common misconceptions about chair yoga for seniors. Providing accurate information and fostering positive experiences will help seniors recognize the value and inclusivity of chair yoga in promoting their overall health and well-being.

"The rhythm of the body, the melody of the mind, and the harmony of the soul create the symphony of life." - B.K.S. Iyengar

CHAPTER THREE

Chair Yoga Weight Loss and Improved Physique

For anyone who want to add light exercise to their routine—including those who are interested in losing weight and toning up—chair yoga can be a helpful and convenient choice.

Even though chair yoga isn't as strenuous as some other types of exercise, it can nevertheless improve general wellbeing and aid with weight control in a number of ways. Here's how to do chair yoga to lose weight and get a better body:

1. **Include Dynamic Chair Yoga Poses:** Take part in resistance-based and movement-based dynamic chair yoga poses. Seated twists, seated forward bends, and seated mountain pose with arm movements are a few examples. These positions encourage strength and flexibility by engaging various muscle groups.

2. Emphasize Core Strengthening: Incorporate postures from chair yoga that work the muscles in the core. The abs and total core stability can be strengthened using sitting leg lifts, seated knee-to-chest stretches, and seated variations of boat posture.

3. Include Cardiovascular Components: Although chair yoga is mostly low-impact, you can include cardiovascular components to increase heart rate and aid with weight loss. Think about including fast-paced chair yoga sequences or adding dynamic exercises like sitting marches and jumping jacks.

4. Use Resistance Bands: To add resistance and strength training to your chair yoga practice, incorporate resistance bands. Exercises like leg lifts with tension bands, bicep curls, and seated rows can improve physique by increasing muscle engagement.

5. **Incorporate postures for Stability and Balance**: Do chair yoga postures that test your stability and balance, like seated tree pose variants, heel-to-toe taps, and side leg lifts. In addition to working the muscles, these poses improve stability overall, which is important for keeping the body in good condition.

6. **Mindful Eating Practices:** Incorporate mindful eating techniques with chair yoga. During meals, practicing mindful awareness can assist you in choosing healthier foods and limiting overindulgence, both of which can aid in managing your weight.

7. **Include Breathing Exercises:** As part of your chair yoga practice, practice breath control, or pranayama. Stress, which is frequently connected to overeating or bad eating habits, can be reduced with the use of deep and conscious breathing techniques.

8. **Practice Frequently**: Reliability is essential. Create a consistent chair yoga practice to get the advantages over time. To encourage weight loss and general health, try to do chair yoga for at least 20 to 30 minutes most days of the week.

9. **Adjust Diet and Lifestyle:** Although chair yoga is a useful part of a healthy lifestyle, it's necessary to combine it with other healthy habits and a balanced diet. For individualized guidance on weight loss, think about speaking with a dietitian or other medical expert.

10. **Remain Hydrated:** Before, during, and after your chair yoga practices, make sure you are well hydrated. Maintaining hydration promotes general health and may help with weight management by enhancing feelings of fullness.

11. **Combine with Other Exercise Forms**: Exercises like walking, swimming, or resistance training can be combined with chair yoga. Combining several exercises can result in a more comprehensive strategy for weight loss and fitness.

12. **Track Progress and Set Objectives:** Keep tabs on your development and make sensible objectives. Having specific goals can help you stay motivated and focused on your fitness path, whether your focus is on strength, flexibility, or general well-being.

Keep in mind that each person may benefit from chair yoga differently when it comes to weight loss and physical enhancement. Speaking with a healthcare provider or fitness specialist is advised, particularly if you have any pre-existing health issues or concerns. Individual outcomes also vary depending on a number of variables, such as lifestyle, nutrition, and general health.

Safety Precautions

When leading chair yoga classes for adults over 60, safety comes first. In light of their distinct requirements and possible health risks, the following crucial safety measures should be observed:

1. **Health Screening**: Perform participant health screenings prior to beginning any chair yoga program. To be sure chair yoga is appropriate for their particular health issues, have them fill out a health questionnaire or speak with a medical specialist.

2. **Individual Assessments**: Perform individual evaluations to learn about the physical capabilities, restrictions, and any particular issues of each participant. This will enable you to modify the chair yoga technique to suit your own needs.

3. **Contact:** Create a clear line of contact with all parties involved. During the session, encourage them to express any pain, discomfort, or worries. Remind them not to push themselves past their comfort zones.

4. **Chair Stability**: Make sure the yoga chairs have a solid foundation and are stable. In order to reduce the possibility of falls or mishaps throughout the exercise, look for any swaying or instability.

5. **Appropriate Seating Position:** Assist participants in adopting the right alignment and posture when sitting. Chairs should be adjusted to provide a straight back and enough back support. Knees should be in line with hips and feet should be flat on the floor.

6. **Accommodations for Participants with Mobility Problems:** Take into account those who may have mobility challenges. Provide adjustments for positions to account for restricted range of motion or difficulties with movement. Promote the use of props for extra support, such as cushions or blocks.

7. **Clearly Stated Instructions**: For every position, give precise, unambiguous instructions. As you lead the participants, model the stances and provide spoken suggestions. Stress how important it is to move mindfully and slowly.

8. **Refrain from Overstretching**: Tell people to stretch only until they experience some minor discomfort, not agony. Injuries can result from overstretching, especially in elderly people who may have less flexibility.

9. **Breathing Awareness**: Stress the need of being aware of your breath. Tell them not to hold their breaths and to breathe comfortably. Breathing slowly and deliberately helps reduce lightheadedness and increase calm.

10. **Individual Assistance:** Be ready to provide help on an individual basis as required. Certain individuals might need further assistance or adjustments. Observe their requirements and adjust your guidance accordingly.

11. **Fall Prevention:** To prevent falls, incorporate balancing exercises using a chair. Encourage participants to practice standing positions with the chair as support, and offer choices for sitting balancing exercises.

12. **Hydration:** Encourage attendees to maintain proper hydration throughout the lesson. In order to avoid dehydration and promote general wellbeing, proper hydration is crucial, particularly for seniors.

13. **Emergency Preparedness**: Learn about emergency protocols and have a backup plan in case something unforeseen occurs. Make sure you know how to use a first aid kit in case you need one and that you have access to one.

14. **Professional assistance:** To make sure you're offering safe and efficient classes, if you're not a trained yoga instructor, think about getting chair yoga certification or assistance, or collaborate with one.

15. **Promote Frequent Check-ins:** Ask participants about their wellbeing on a regular basis. To make the chair yoga sessions even better, promote candid discussion and solicit input.

You may provide elders practicing chair yoga with a safe and encouraging setting by putting these safety measures into practice. Keep in mind that each participant is different, and customized care and modifications are essential to guaranteeing a secure and pleasurable event for all parties.

"Yoga is the fountain of youth. You're only as young as your spine is flexible." - Bob Harper

Ideal Chairs and Additional Props
Needed for Chair Yoga for seniors

Senior chair yoga sessions can be conducted safely and effectively by selecting the appropriate chair and adding extra props. Here are some tips for choosing the perfect chair and ideas for extra props:

1. **Sturdy and Stable**: Select a chair that is both stable and robust. To ensure everyone's safety — especially those who might require additional support — it should not sway or have loose sections.

2. **Armless and Straight Back:** To provide a complete range of motion, choose a chair without arms. When seated, a straight-backed chair with a firm seat is the best choice for encouraging good posture.

3. **Flat Seat:** Verify that the chair's seat is level and flat. This lessens discomfort during the

exercise and aids in maintaining correct alignment for the participants.

4. **Comfortable Seat Cushion:** If the chair's seat is excessively firm, think about adding a cushion. This can improve comfort, particularly for elderly people who are sensitive or uneasy in a sitting position.

5. **Adjustable Height:** Look for a chair that can be adjusted in height if at all possible. This enables you to adjust the chair's height to meet each participant's unique demands.

6. **Non-Slip Surface:** To avoid any sliding or movement during poses, make sure the chair has a non-slip surface. This is crucial for stability, especially when standing or doing balance postures.

Extra Credits:

1. **Yoga Blocks**: You may adjust poses with yoga blocks, which also offer extra support and

help with alignment. They are especially beneficial for people who have restricted range of motion or flexibility.

2. **Cushions or Bolsters:** Participants experiencing lower back discomfort may find that additional support is provided by cushions or bolsters. For added comfort, place pillows between the thighs or beneath the knees when in seated positions.

3. **Resistance Bands:** Chair yoga gains a strength training component with the use of resistance bands. They can be used to create muscle strength through seated exercises that work the arms, shoulders, and legs while offering mild resistance.

4. **Tiny Blanket**: When assuming relaxation positions, a tiny blanket can be utilized to enhance comfort. For warmth and support, participants can drape the blanket over their laps or shoulders.

5. **Strap or Belt**: For people who might have trouble reaching their hands or feet, straps or belts can be helpful. They can be used to increase reach in specific postures and stretches.

6. **Stability Ball:** To strengthen your core and enhance your balance, try some seated workouts with a stability ball. It increases the degree of instability, which prompts participants to use their stabilizing muscles.

7. **Hand Weights (Optional):** Hand weights can be used during sitting exercises to increase arm and shoulder strength for those seeking to undertake light resistance training. Make sure the weights are suitable for each person's level of fitness.

8. **Tennis balls or massage balls**: You can self-massage and relieve tension in different areas of your body by using tennis balls or massage

balls. They work especially well for mild myofascial release.

9. **Chair Yoga DVD or Online Videos**: If you're looking for guided practices, think about investing in a chair yoga DVD or online videos. Participants can use this to reinforce what they've learnt in class and carry out their practice at home.

When introducing props, make sure to give participants precise information on how to use them and encourage them to use them as required for support and comfort. Furthermore, pay close attention to each participant's unique demands and provide adjustments or substitutes as needed. Senior chair yoga classes must be successful in fostering a safe and welcoming environment.

Perfect Setting for an Enjoyable Practice
Senior chair yoga requires careful consideration of both the physical area and the general ambiance to create a perfect and comfortable space. Here's a checklist to assist you in creating a warm and inviting environment:

Physical Area:

1. **Sufficient Lighting**: Make sure there is enough natural or soft lighting in the area. In addition to being crucial for safety, adequate lighting also fosters a cozy and welcoming ambiance.

2. **Open and Uncluttered Area:** Make sure the area is free of clutter and impediments to allow for easy mobility. Seniors in particular may require additional room and well-defined routes during the exercise.

3. **Non-Slip Flooring**: To avoid any unintentional slips or falls, especially during

standing or balance poses, use a non-slip floor or install non-slip mats below chairs.

4. **Comfy Seating Configuration:** Position seats such that everyone can move around easily and see each other. To prevent crowding, make sure that every chair is appropriately spaced.

5. **Appropriate Ventilation:** Make sure the space has adequate ventilation. Comfort requires adequate ventilation, particularly when engaging in vigorous activity. Open doors or windows to let in fresh air if available.

6. **Comfortable Temperature:** Make sure the room is at a temperature that is cozy. To ensure that participants can concentrate on the practice without being distracted, the environment shouldn't be excessively hot or chilly.

7. **Calm and Quiet Ambience:** Reduce outside disturbances and cultivate a calm and peaceful ambiance. If you can, practice chair yoga in a quiet place to improve its meditative qualities.

8. **Accessible Restrooms:** For the comfort of participants, make sure accessible restrooms are close by. Seniors who might need to use the facilities during the program should pay particular attention to this.

9. **Atmosphere:**

i. *Warm and Welcome Decor:* Furnish the area with items that exude warmth and welcome. For added ambience, think about adding artwork, plants, or soothing hues.

ii. *Calm Music or Nature Sounds:* To create a peaceful atmosphere, play mellow instrumental music or natural sounds. Make sure the volume is just low enough to be background noise without becoming annoying.

iii. *Aromatherapy:* Take into account employing fragrant candles or essential oils for delicate aromatherapy. Aromas like chamomile or lavender can improve the atmosphere and aid in relaxation.

iv. *Personalized Touches:* To create a welcoming atmosphere, add personalized touches. This could include blankets, pillows, or any other furnishings that help create a warm and inviting space.

v. *Establish a Focal Point:* Choose a focal point, like a stunning work of art or a soothing picture. This can be used as a focal point when practicing relaxation techniques or meditation.

vi. *Promote Social Interaction*: Promoting social interaction will help to build a feeling of community. Establish a welcoming and inclusive location where participants can congregate both before and after the program.

vii. *Offer Refreshments*: Before or after the session, think about providing water or herbal tea. Maintaining proper hydration is crucial, and a modest refreshment station is a considerate addition.

viii. *Establish a Calm Entry Experience:* Give careful thought to the entry experience. Make sure everyone is made to feel at home as soon as they arrive. To set the mood, think about adding a welcome sign, dim lighting, or soothing music.

ix. *Community-Supportive Atmosphere*: Encourage a community-focused and supportive environment. In order to foster a sense of unity within the group, encourage people to ask questions, share their experiences, and so on.

x. *Clear Instruction and Encouragement:* Establish a good mood by giving directions that are both clear and encouraging. Establish a space where people can feel encouraged and that their efforts are valued.

Chair yoga for seniors can be practiced in the perfect environment if the physical space and general ambience are carefully considered. An environment that is welcoming and pleasant improves the whole experience, making it more pleasurable and beneficial to participants' well-being.

Setting up for success in Chair Yoga
Setting up for success in chair yoga involves careful planning, thoughtful consideration of participants' needs, and creating a positive and inclusive atmosphere. Here's a guide to help you establish a successful chair yoga session:

1. Understand Your Participants:

Conduct Health Assessments: Prior to the sessions, gather information about participants' health conditions, mobility levels, and any specific concerns. This will help you tailor the chair yoga practice to meet their individual needs.

2. Choose the Right Venue:

Accessible Space: Select a space that is accessible and accommodating for seniors. Ensure there's enough room for participants to move comfortably, and the environment is free of obstacles.

3. **Provide Comfortable Seating:**

Choose Appropriate Chairs: Ensure that chairs are sturdy, armless, and have a firm seat. Consider adding cushions for extra comfort. Check for any wobbling or instability to guarantee the safety of participants.

4. **Set Up the Space:**

Clear Pathways: Arrange chairs in a way that allows for clear pathways and easy movement. Remove any obstacles or hazards to create a safe environment.

5. **Create a Relaxing Atmosphere:**

Adequate Lighting: Use soft, natural, or warm lighting to create a calming atmosphere. Consider incorporating lamps or candles for a serene ambiance.

Background Music or Nature Sounds: Play gentle instrumental music or nature sounds at a low volume to enhance relaxation. Ensure it complements the practice without being distracting.

6. Provide Necessary Props:

- *Yoga Blocks*: Have yoga blocks for modifications and additional support.

- *Cushions or Bolsters*: Offer cushions or bolsters for added comfort, especially for those with lower back discomfort.

- *Resistance Bands:* Integrate resistance bands for strength training.

- *Straps or Belts*: Provide straps or belts for participants who may need assistance with reaching.

- *Small Blankets:* Have small blankets for relaxation poses.

7. Educate and Communicate:

Orientation Session: Conduct an orientation session to educate participants about chair yoga, its benefits, and what to expect. Address any concerns or questions they may have.

Clear Instructions: During the session, provide clear and concise instructions for each pose. Demonstrate poses when necessary and use verbal cues to guide participants.

8. Encourage Participation:

Promote Inclusivity: Create an inclusive environment where participants feel comfortable and supported. Encourage everyone to participate at their own pace and provide modifications for different fitness levels.

Acknowledge Efforts: Acknowledge participants' efforts and progress. Positive reinforcement fosters a sense of accomplishment and motivates continued participation.

9. Ensure Safety:

Monitor Participants: Pay close attention to participants' movements and provide individual assistance when needed. Be vigilant for signs of discomfort or fatigue.

Emergency Preparedness: Familiarize yourself with emergency procedures and have access to a first aid kit. Ensure participants are aware of emergency exits and procedures.

10. **Promote Social Interaction:**

Community Building: Foster a sense of community by providing opportunities for social interaction before or after sessions. Encourage participants to share their experiences and build connections.

11. **Variety in Sessions:**

Diverse Sessions: Offer a variety of chair yoga sessions, including sessions focused on flexibility, strength, balance, and relaxation. This ensures a well-rounded experience for participants.

12. **Gather Feedback:**

Feedback Mechanism: Establish a feedback mechanism to gather input from participants. This can help you understand their preferences, address concerns, and continuously improve the chair yoga sessions.

By carefully considering the needs of your participants, creating a conducive environment, and fostering a positive atmosphere, you set the stage for success in chair yoga sessions. Regularly assess and adjust your approach based on feedback and evolving participant needs to ensure ongoing success and participant satisfaction.

"Yoga is a light, which once lit, will never dim. The better your practice, the brighter the flame." - B.K.S. Iyengar

CHAPTER FOUR

Basic Chair Yoga Poses

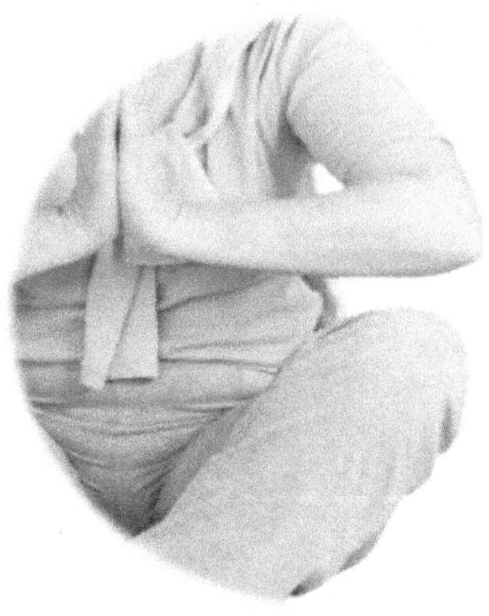

Simple chair yoga positions that you can include in your practice. The goals of these poses are to increase *strength, flexibility, and calmness*. Encourage participants to move sensibly and comfortably at all times. Safety should always come first, and participants should always remember to speak with their healthcare providers if they have any health concerns.

1. **Seated Mountain Pose**:

   - Sit with your feet flat on the floor and your spine straight.
   - Plant hands on knees or thighs.
   - Exhale, extend your back, and raise your arms in the air.
   - Let go and lower your arms again.

2. **Forward Bend While Seated**:

   - Place your feet flat on the floor.
   - Breathe in and extend your spine.
   - Let out a breath, turn your hips, and extend your hands to your shins or the ground.

> Hold for a short while.

3. Seated Twist:

> Sit upright on your chair.
> Breathe in and extend your spine.
> Release your breath, turn to the side, and place one hand on the knee across from you and the other on the chair's back.
> Take a few deep breaths, hold, and then switch to the other side.

4. Seated Cat-Cow Stretch:

> Maintain a straight back when sitting.
> Take a breath, lift your chest, and arch your back.
> Exhale, arch your back, and rest your chin on your chest.
> Continue, switching between the cow and cat stretches.

5. Side stretch while seated:

> Place your feet flat on the floor.
> Breathe in and extend your spine.

- Lean to one side, let out a breath, and raise one arm overhead.
- Take a few deep breaths, hold, and then switch to the other side.

Extra Advice: - Breathing: Instruct participants to match their motions to calm, deep breaths.

- *Calm Motions:* Stress the value of calm, deliberate motions; steer clear of any abrupt or violent movements.

- *Comfort*: Tell participants to take a comfortable seat, and if necessary, use cushions or other props.

- *Modify as Needed:* Participants are welcome to adjust poses to suit their degree of comfort and any physical restrictions.

These fundamental chair yoga positions can be modified for certain purposes or combined into a short sequence. More poses and variations can be added gradually as participants get more at ease. Remind participants that chair yoga is about finding joy and relaxation in movement, and always foster an inclusive and friendly environment.

6. **Warrior Pose in Sitting**:

> ➢ Place your feet hip-width apart.
> ➢ With the foot flexed, extend one leg forward.
> ➢ Take a breath and lift both arms high.
> ➢ Switch legs after holding for a few breaths.

7. **Seated Butterfly Stretch**:

> ➢ Bend your knees outward while sitting with your feet together.
> ➢ Remain upright while bending your knees slightly toward the floor.
> ➢ A mild elasticity in the inner thighs is sensed.

8. **Sitting Pigeon Pose**:

> ➢ Take a seat on the chair's edge.

- ➢ Fold one ankle over the knee of the other.
- ➢ Maintain a straight back while bending slightly forward to feel your outer hip stretch.
- ➢ Continue on the opposite side.

9. **Seated Chest Opener:**

- ➢ Maintain a straight back when sitting.
- ➢ Straighten your arms and clasp your hands behind your back.
- ➢ Squeeze the shoulder blades together while raising the chest and opening the shoulders.

10. **Seated Eagle Arms:**

- ➢ Maintain a straight back while sitting.
- ➢ Place one arm across the other so that the palms meet.
- ➢ Raise elbows to shoulder level so that your upper back feels stretched.
- ➢ Continue by placing the other arm on top.

11. **Seated Ankle Rolls**:

> ➤ Raise one foot off the floor and give the ankle a mild 360-degree spin.
> ➤ Change to your other foot.

12. **Side leg lifts while seated:**

> ➤ Place your feet flat on the floor.
> ➤ Raise one leg to the side so that the outside thigh is involved.
> ➤ Lower, then switch to the opposite side.

13. **Sun Salutation while seated:**

> ➤ Take a breath, raise your arms.
> ➤ Let go and place your hands over your hearts.
> ➤ Take a breath and raise your arms above your head.
> ➤ Let go, turn your hips, and extend your arm forward.
> ➤ Take a breath, extend your back.
> ➤ Let out a breath and return to the beginning posture.

14. **Seated Tree Pose:**

> - Sit upright in a chair.
> - Elevate one foot and press the sole against the opposing leg's inner thigh or calf.
> - Raise your hands to your hearts.
> - Hold, then switch to the other leg.

15. **Arms in the Seated Cow Face Pose:**

> - Raise your right arm, bend your elbow, and put your hand down your back.
> - Try to clasp fingers by reaching behind the left arm.
> - Place a strap or towel between the hands if they are not meeting.

Extra Advice:

Flowing Sequences: For a dynamic chair yoga practice, combine these positions into flowing sequences.

Mindful Awareness: Throughout the activity, remind participants to pay attention to their breath and bodily sensations.

Creative Expression: Within the parameters of comfort and safety, allow participants to experiment and express themselves.

You can easily modify these poses to fit your participants' needs and adjust the routine to fit their skill level and preferences. One adaptable and easily accessible technique to reap the advantages of yoga while seated is through chair yoga.

16. **Seated Knee Hug**:

> Maintain a straight back when sitting.
> Holding onto the shin, give one knee a hug towards the chest.
> After a few breaths of holding, switch legs.

17. **Sitting Hamstring Stretch**:

> Straighten one leg while keeping the heel on the ground.
> Breathe in and extend your spine.

> Breathe out, swivel at the hips, and
  extend your reach to your toes.
> Switch legs after holding for a few
  breaths.

18. **In-seated biceps:**

> Sit with your feet flat on the ground to
  stretch.
> Lift one foot while holding the ankle
  toward the buttocks.
> The front of the thigh should feel
  stretched.
> Grab and rotate your legs.

19. **Figure 4 Stretch while Seated:**

> Place your feet flat on the floor.
> Fold one ankle over the knee of the other.
> To increase the stretch's depth, lightly
  press on the crossed knee.
> Continue on the opposite side.

20. **Seated Side Leg Stretch:**

> Extend your legs wide while sitting.

- ➢ Breathe in and extend your spine.
- ➢ Release your breath, reach for one foot, and feel your body being stretched down the side.
- ➢ After a few breaths of holding, switch sides.

21. **Seated High Altar Twist:**

- ➢ Maintain a straight back while sitting.
- ➢ Exhale and lift your arms skyward.
- ➢ Let out a breath, turn to the side, and place one hand on the knee across from you and the other hand behind the chair.
- ➢ After a few breaths of holding, switch sides.

22. **Half Moon Pose in Sitting:**

- ➢ Sit upright.
- ➢ Raise one arm overhead and stretch to the other side.
- ➢ Sensate a stretch down the body's side.

> After a few breaths of holding, switch sides.

23. **Sitting Hip Opener:**

   - Place your feet flat on the floor.
   - Fold one ankle over the knee of the other.
   - To open the hip, gently press on the crossed knee.
   - Continue on the opposite side.

24. **Seated Eagle Leg:**

   - Place the foot under the calf and cross one leg over the other.
   - Switch legs after holding for a few breaths.

25. **Garland sat Position:**

   - Take a seat at the chair's edge, placing your feet flat on the floor.
   - Spread the knees wide and converge the toes of the feet.
   - While holding the feet, budge the knees slightly toward the floor.

Extra Advice: -

Chair Yoga Flow: Mix these positions to create a flowing sequence that encourages practitioners to move fluidly from one pose to the next.

Breath Awareness: Encourage participants to move in time with their breathing to promote calmness and mindfulness.

Personal Exploration: Encourage individuals to experiment with the positions, finding what feels good for their bodies and modifying them to suit.

To construct a well-rounded and fun chair yoga regimen, feel free to mix and match these positions. As usual, modify the poses to suit each participant's needs and remind them to pay attention to their body during the practice.

26. **Warrior II in the Seat:**

> ➢ Place your feet wide apart.

- Extend your arms parallel to the floor and turn one foot outward.
- Feel a slight stretch in the inner thigh as you look over the front hand.
- Continue on the opposite side.

27. Seated Warrior III:

- Sit upright in your chair.
- Straighten one leg and extend it back, maintaining the toes on the ground.
- Reach forward, keeping your arms parallel to the floor.
- Switch legs after holding for a few breaths.

28. Seated Side Plank:

- Maintain a straight back when sitting.
- Lift your hips, place one hand on the chair, and reach up toward the ceiling with your other arm.
- After a few breaths of holding, switch sides.

29. **Seated Boat Pose**:

> ➤ Sit upright in a chair.
> ➤ Elevate your legs off the ground while maintaining your sit bones.
> ➤ Stretch your arms outward, parallel to the floor.
> ➤ Hold for a short while.

30. **Seated Lunge**:

> ➤ Take a seat at the chair's edge.
> ➤ Raise one leg back and droop your hips a little.
> ➤ The front of the hip should feel stretched.
> ➤ After a few breaths of holding, switch legs.

31. **Straighten your back while sitting in the camel pose:**

> ➤ Lay hands with fingers pointing down on lower back.
> ➤ Taking a breath, raise your chest, and softly arch your spine back.
> ➤ Take a couple breaths and hold.

32. **Twisted Mountain Pose**:

➢ Sit with your back to the chair.
➢ Take a breath and raise your arms.
➢ Let out a breath, turn to the side, and place one hand on the knee across from you and the other hand behind the chair.
➢ After a few breaths of holding, switch sides.

33. **Seated Reverse Plank:**

➢ Maintain a straight back while sitting.
➢ With your fingers pointed toward your feet, place your hands on the chair.
➢ Raise your hips so that your head and heels are in a straight line.
➢ Hold for a short while.

34. **Leaning Leg Cross Twist:**

➢ Sit upright in your chair.
➢ Twist toward the crossed knee while crossing one leg over the other.

> After a few breaths of holding, switch sides.

35. **Garland seated Pose Variation**:

> Spread your feet apart and sit at the chair's edge. Press elbows against inner knees and raise hands to the center of the heart.
> Take a couple breaths and hold.

Extra Advice:

Flowing Transitions: Motivate participants to move fluidly between poses while keeping their breath in mind.

Balancing Poses: As participants gain stability and confidence, introduce increasingly difficult sitting balancing poses.

Individual Exploration: Encourage people to experiment with different versions and personalize the poses to fit their own needs and comfort zones.

The chair yoga sequences can be adjusted and changed according to the skills and preferences of the participants. Remind participants that the goal of the exercise is to find calm and joy in movement, and encourage them to listen to their bodies.

"Age is not a limit to fitness; it's a state of mind."

CHAPTER FIVE

Gentle Stretches for Flexibility

Neck Stretches

Instructions

- o Sit comfortably with a tall spine.
- o Inhale, lengthen your neck, and as you exhale, gently tilt your head to one side, bringing your ear toward your shoulder.
- o Hold the stretch for a few breaths, feeling the gentle stretch along the side of your neck.
- o Inhale to return to the center and repeat on the other side.
- o You can also add variations like nodding your head forward and backward.

Benefits

- o Relieves tension in the neck and shoulders.
- o Improves flexibility and range of motion in the neck.
- o Promotes relaxation.

Shoulder Rolls
Instructions

- o Sit comfortably with your hands on your thighs.
- o Inhale, lift your shoulders towards your ears.
- o Exhale, roll your shoulders back and down in a circular motion.
- o Repeat this movement for several rounds and then reverse the direction.
- o Focus on keeping the movements smooth and controlled.

Benefits

- o Releases tension in the shoulders and upper back.
- o Improves flexibility and mobility in the shoulder joints.
- o Enhances circulation in the upper body.

Instructions

- o Extend your arms in front of you with palms facing down.
- o Rotate your wrists in circular motions, first in one direction and then the other.
- o Open and close your fists, stretching your fingers wide and then making a fist.
- o Repeat these exercises for a few rounds, paying attention to any sensations in your wrists and hands.

Benefits

- o Increases flexibility in the wrists and fingers.
- o Alleviates stiffness in the hands and wrists.
- o Promotes joint health.

Instructions

- o Sit with your feet flat on the floor.
- o Lift one foot and rotate your ankle in a circular motion, first clockwise and then counterclockwise.
- o Point and flex your toes, moving your foot in various directions.
- o Repeat on the other foot.
- o For toe flexibility, try spreading your toes wide and then squeezing them together.

Benefits

- o Improves flexibility and range of motion in the ankles.
- o Strengthens the muscles around the ankles and toes.
- o Enhances balance and stability.

Additional Tips:

- *Mindful Breathing:* Throughout these stretches, encourage participants to focus on their breath. Inhale deeply during the preparatory phase and exhale as they move into the stretch. This enhances relaxation and mindfulness.

- *Gradual Progression:* Remind participants to move gradually and avoid pushing themselves into discomfort. Flexibility improves with consistent practice, so encourage regular participation.

- *Individual Adaptations*: Emphasize that these stretches can be adapted to individual needs and comfort levels. Participants should feel free to modify the intensity of the stretches based on their own flexibility and any existing health conditions.

"Yoga is invigoration in relaxation. Freedom in routine. Confidence through self-control. Energy within and energy without." - Ymber Delecto

CHAPTER SIX

Chair Yoga for Strength

Seated Leg Lifts
Instructions

- o Sit comfortably with your back straight and feet flat on the floor.
- o Lift one leg straight out in front of you, engaging the thigh muscles.
- o Hold the leg in the lifted position for a few breaths.
- o Lower the leg back down and repeat on the other side.
- o For added challenge, lift both legs simultaneously.

Benefits

- o Strengthens the quadriceps and thigh muscles.
- o Improves stability and balance.
- o Engages the core muscles.

Chair Squats
Instructions

- o Stand behind the chair with feet hip-width apart.

o Inhale, engage your core, and as you exhale, lower your body into a seated position as if you were sitting in the chair.
o Keep your knees aligned with your toes and your weight in your heels.
o Inhale to stand back up, squeezing your glutes at the top.
o Repeat for several repetitions.

Benefits

o Strengthens the quadriceps, hamstrings, and glutes.
o Targets the core muscles.
o Improves lower body endurance.

Arm Exercises with Resistance Bands
Instructions

o Sit or stand with the resistance band securely anchored.
o Hold the ends of the band in your hands.

- o Perform exercises such as bicep curls, shoulder presses, or lateral raises using the resistance band.
- o Control the movement both on the way up and on the way down.

Benefits

- o Builds strength in the biceps, triceps, and shoulder muscles.
- o Enhances overall arm strength and tone.
- o Offers resistance for increased muscle engagement.
- o

Core Strengthening Poses

a. **Seated Boat Pose**

- o Sit on the edge of the chair with your back straight.
- o Hold onto the sides of the chair and lift your legs off the ground, balancing on your sit bones.
- o Engage your core and hold the position for a few breaths.

- o Lower your feet back to the ground.

b. **Seated Russian Twists**

- o Sit with your back straight and knees bent.
- o Hold onto the sides of the chair and lean back slightly.
- o Twist your torso to one side, then the other, engaging your obliques.
- o Repeat the twisting motion for several rounds.

Benefits

- o Strengthens the abdominal muscles.
- o Improves core stability and balance.
- o Targets the muscles of the back and obliques.

Additional Tips

- *Proper Form:* Emphasize the importance of maintaining proper form during each exercise. Participants should focus on controlled movements to avoid strain or injury.

- *Breathing*: Instruct participants to synchronize their breath with the movements. Encourage deep inhalations during the preparatory phase and exhalations during the exertion phase.

- *Modify Intensity:* Participants can modify the intensity of the exercises based on their fitness level. It's essential to find a balance between challenge and comfort.

- *Consistency*: Encourage regular practice to see improvements in strength over time. Consistency is key for building and maintaining muscle strength.

CHAPTER SEVEN
Balance and Stability Exercises

Seated Knee Lifts
Instructions

- o Sit comfortably with your back straight and feet flat on the floor.
- o Lift one knee toward your chest, keeping the foot hovering above the ground.
- o Hold the position for a few breaths, engaging your core for stability.
- o Lower the foot back down and repeat on the other side.
- o For added challenge, lift both knees simultaneously.

Benefits

- o Improves hip flexor strength.
- o Enhances core stability.
- o Focuses on balance and coordination

Heel-to-Toe Taps
Instructions

- o Sit on the edge of the chair with your feet flat on the floor.
- o Lift one foot and tap the heel on the floor in front of you.
- o Return the foot to the starting position.
- o Repeat the movement with the other foot.
- o Alternate between heel taps for several repetitions.

Benefits

- o Enhances ankle flexibility and mobility.
- o Improves coordination and balance.
- o Engages muscles in the lower legs.

Modified Tree Pose
Instructions

o Sit with your back straight and feet flat on the floor.
o Lift one foot off the ground and place the sole against the inner thigh or calf of the opposite leg.
o Find your balance and bring your palms together at the chest in a prayer position.
o Hold the position for a few breaths and then switch to the other leg.

Benefits

o Increases hip flexibility.
o Develops anklc stability.
o Challenges balance and concentration.

Balancing on One Leg
Instructions

o Stand behind the chair with feet hip-width apart.
o Hold onto the back of the chair for support.

o Lift one leg off the ground, bending the knee.
o Find your balance and hold the position for a few breaths.
o Lower the foot back down and switch to the other leg.

Benefits

o Strengthens the muscles around the ankles and calves.
o Improves overall balance and stability.
o Enhances proprioception (awareness of body position in space).

Additional Tips:

Focus on a Point: Encourage participants to find a focal point to gaze at during balancing exercises. This helps with concentration and balance.

Use Props: Participants can use the chair for added support during these exercises.

Gradually, as their balance improves, they can decrease reliance on the chair.

Safety First: Emphasize the importance of safety. Participants should perform these exercises in a safe environment, and they should hold onto the chair or a stable surface if needed.

Progress Gradually: Progression in balance exercises may take time. Participants should gradually increase the duration and intensity of these exercises as their stability improves.

"Your body exists in the past and your mind exists in the future. In yoga, they come together in the present." - B.K.S. Iyengar

CHAPTER EIGHT
Relaxation and Breathing Techniques

Deep Breathing Exercises
Instructions

- o Sit comfortably with your back straight and shoulders relaxed.
- o Inhale deeply through your nose, expanding your diaphragm.
- o Exhale slowly and completely through your mouth or nose.
- o Focus on making your breaths smooth, deep, and rhythmic.
- o Gradually extend the duration of inhalation and exhalation.

Benefits

- o Calms the nervous system.
- o Reduces stress and anxiety.
- o Improves lung capacity and respiratory function.

Guided Relaxation
Instructions

o Sit or recline comfortably in the chair.
o Close your eyes and bring awareness to your breath.
o Inhale deeply and exhale fully, letting go of tension.
o Guide participants through a relaxation script, focusing on each part of the body.
o Encourage them to visualize a peaceful scene or engage their senses in a calming way.

Benefits

o Induces a state of deep relaxation.
o Releases physical and mental tension.
o Promotes a sense of inner peace and tranquility.

Meditation in a Chair
Instructions

- o Sit comfortably with your back straight and hands resting on your lap.
- o Close your eyes or maintain a soft gaze.
- o Focus on your breath or a chosen point of concentration.
- o Allow thoughts to come and go without attachment.
- o Practice mindfulness by bringing attention back to the present moment.

Benefits

- o Enhances mental clarity and focus.
- o Reduces stress and promotes emotional well-being.
- o Cultivates a sense of mindfulness and self-awareness.

Additional Tips:

- Mindful Body Scan: During guided relaxation, encourage participants to perform a mindful body scan, bringing awareness to each part of the body and consciously releasing tension.

- Use Relaxing Imagery: Incorporate imagery that resonates with relaxation, such as visualizing a peaceful beach, a serene forest, or a gentle stream. The power of suggestion can deepen the relaxation experience.

- Silent Meditation: In guided meditation, allow moments of silent meditation where participants can explore their inner stillness without external guidance. This allows for a more personal and introspective experience.

- Comfortable Seating: Ensure that participants are seated in a comfortable and supportive chair. If needed, provide cushions or blankets for additional comfort during relaxation and meditation.

- Encourage Regular Practice: Emphasize the importance of regular practice of relaxation and breathing techniques. Consistent practice can lead to long-term benefits in managing stress and promoting overall well-being.

Relaxation and breathing techniques play a pivotal role in chair yoga, offering participants the opportunity to unwind, release tension, and connect with a sense of inner calm. As an instructor, your guidance and encouragement create a nurturing space for participants to experience the profound benefits of relaxation and mindfulness. Always adapt these techniques to suit the comfort and preferences of your participants, fostering a supportive and peaceful environment.

CHAPTER NINE

Chair Yoga Routines

Below is a detailed and comprehensive note on chair yoga routines for different times of the day—morning, afternoon, and evening.

Morning Chair Yoga Routine

Objective: Energize the body, promote flexibility, and set a positive tone for the day.

1. **Seated Mountain Pose**

   - Inhale and reach arms overhead.

   - Stretch the spine and engage core muscles.

   - Exhale and lower arms.

2. **Seated Forward Bend**

   - Inhale, lengthen the spine.

   - Exhale, hinge at the hips, reaching towards toes.

   - Hold and breathe deeply.

3. **Seated Twist**

   - Inhale, lengthen the spine.

   - Exhale, twist to one side, holding the back of the chair.

   - Repeat on the other side.

4. **Seated Knee Lifts**

   - Lift knees towards the chest.

   - Engage the core and hold briefly.

   - Lower legs and repeat.

5. **Deep Breathing Exercises**

   - Perform deep breathing exercises for 3-5 minutes.

   - Inhale through the nose, exhale through the mouth.

6. **Arm Circles**

   - Extend arms to the sides.

- Rotate arms in circular motions, forward and backward.

7. Morning Meditation

- Guide participants through a short morning meditation focusing on gratitude and positive intentions for the day.

Closing:

- Encourage participants to maintain a positive mindset throughout the day.

- Remind them to carry the benefits of the morning practice with them.

Afternoon Stretch Break

Objective: Release tension, improve focus, and boost energy levels.

1. Chair Squats

- Stand and perform chair squats.

- Inhale to lower, exhale to stand.

2. Heel-to-Toe Taps:

   - Sit on the edge of the chair.

   - Lift and tap heels on the floor.

3. Wrist and Hand Exercises:

   - Perform exercises to release tension in wrists and hands.

4. Seated Cat-Cow Stretch:

   - Sit tall and perform seated cat-cow stretches.

5. Guided Relaxation:

   - Sit comfortably and guide participants through a brief relaxation focusing on letting go of afternoon stress.

6. Deep Breathing Break:

   - Engage in deep breathing exercises for relaxation and reenergizing.

7. Neck and Shoulder Stretches:

   - Perform gentle neck and shoulder stretches.

Closing:

   - Encourage participants to take short stretch breaks throughout the afternoon.

   - Emphasize the importance of mindful movement for mental clarity.

Evening Relaxation Sequence
Objective: Wind down, release tension, and promote restful sleep.

1. Seated Side Stretch:

   - Inhale and lift one arm, stretching to the side.

   - Exhale and repeat on the other side.

2. Seated Boat Pose:

- Lift legs off the ground, engaging core.

- Hold the position for a few breaths.

3. Balancing on One Leg:

- Stand and balance on one leg with support.

- Switch to the other leg.

4. Guided Relaxation:

- Perform a longer guided relaxation, focusing on each part of the body.

5. Evening Meditation:

- Guide participants through a calming evening meditation to prepare for sleep.

6. Deep Breathing for Sleep:

- Practice deep breathing exercises with an emphasis on relaxation.

7. Closing Thoughts:

- Encourage participants to reflect on positive aspects of their day.

- Suggest carrying a sense of calm into bedtime routine.

Additional Tips:

- Adaptations: Encourage participants to adapt the routines based on their comfort and abilities.

- Consistency: Stress the importance of consistent practice for maximum benefits.

- Individual Pace: Remind participants to move at their own pace and listen to their bodies.

CHAPTER TEN

Adapting Chair Yoga for Individual needs

Adapting chair yoga for individual needs is crucial to ensure inclusivity and safety for participants with varying abilities, mobility issues, or chronic conditions. Here's a well-detailed note on adapting chair yoga:

Modifying Poses for Mobility Issues
Considerations

- Individual Assessment: Begin by assessing each participant's mobility and flexibility. This allows you to understand their specific needs and limitations.

- Range of Motion: Modify poses to accommodate limited range of motion. For example, reduce the height of arm movements or limit the range of a twist.

- Chair Support: Encourage participants to use the chair for support, especially during standing poses. The chair provides stability and reduces the risk of falls.

Examples of Modifications

- Seated Mountain Pose: If reaching arms overhead is challenging, participants can keep hands on thighs or at heart center.

- Seated Forward Bend: Adapt by allowing participants to bend their knees or only reach as far as comfortable.

- Chair Squats: Adjust the depth of the squat based on participants' comfort level.

Chair Yoga for Those with Chronic Conditions
Considerations

- Health History Assessment: Collect detailed information about participants' chronic conditions, medications, and any restrictions provided by their healthcare professionals.

- Low-Impact Options: Choose poses and exercises that are low-impact and gentle on joints. Focus on improving mobility without exacerbating existing conditions.

- Breathing Emphasis: Incorporate breathing exercises, as controlled breathing can help manage symptoms associated with chronic conditions.

Examples of Adaptations:

- Breathing Exercises: Emphasize slow, deep breathing to promote relaxation and reduce stress.

- Gentle Stretches: Modify stretches for comfort, ensuring participants can control the intensity.

- Supported Poses: Use props like cushions or blocks to provide additional support during poses.

Consulting with a Healthcare Professional
Considerations:

- Encourage Consultation: Urge participants to consult with their healthcare professionals before starting a chair yoga program, especially if they have chronic conditions or are unsure about their fitness level.

- Share Program Details: Provide healthcare professionals with details about the chair yoga program, including the types of poses, intensity, and duration. This ensures that they can offer guidance tailored to the individual's health status.

- Open Communication: Maintain open communication with participants and encourage them to communicate any changes in their health or concerns. This information can guide further adaptations as needed.

Benefits of Consulting with Healthcare Professionals

- Personalized Guidance: Healthcare professionals can offer personalized recommendations based on individual health needs.

- Safety Assurance: Ensures that participants engage in chair yoga safely, minimizing the risk of exacerbating existing conditions.

- Optimal Support: Collaboration between yoga instructors and healthcare professionals provides optimal support for participants' overall well-being.

Additional Tips:

- Inclusive Language: Use inclusive language that acknowledges and respects participants' diverse abilities and conditions.

- Continuous Communication: Maintain an open line of communication with participants, encouraging them to share any discomfort or concerns during sessions.

- Provide Options: Offer variations and options for poses, allowing participants to choose what feels comfortable for them.

- Regular Check-Ins: Periodically check in with participants to assess their comfort level and any changes in their condition.

Adapting chair yoga for individual needs is a thoughtful and dynamic process that requires continuous communication, flexibility, and a commitment to ensuring the well-being of all participants. By fostering a supportive and inclusive environment, chair yoga can be a beneficial practice for individuals with various abilities and health conditions.

CHAPTER ELEVEN

Frequently Asked Questions about Chair Yoga

Can I do Chair Yoga with existing health conditions?

Absolutely, chair yoga can be adapted to accommodate various health conditions. However, it's essential to consult with your healthcare professional before starting a chair yoga practice, especially if you have existing health concerns. They can provide personalized guidance based on your specific health situation, ensuring that chair yoga is safe and beneficial for you.

Considerations:

- Health Assessment: Understand your health condition and inform your yoga instructor about any restrictions or concerns.

- Modification of Poses: Chair yoga poses can be modified to suit different needs. Your instructor can provide variations or suggest alternative poses to ensure comfort and safety.

- Communication: Regularly communicate with your healthcare professional and yoga instructor about any changes in your health or symptoms. This helps in adapting the practice as needed.

How often should I practice Chair Yoga?
The frequency of chair yoga practice can vary based on individual preferences, schedules, and health conditions. Generally, starting with 2-3 sessions per week is a good approach. Regular, consistent practice is more beneficial than infrequent intense sessions.

Considerations:

- Personal Schedule: Find a frequency that fits into your daily or weekly routine comfortably.

- Gradual Progression: If you're new to chair yoga, start with shorter sessions and gradually increase the duration as your comfort and confidence grow.

- Listen to Your Body: Pay attention to how your body responds. If you experience fatigue or discomfort, consider adjusting the frequency or intensity of your practice.

Are there any age restrictions for Chair Yoga?
Chair yoga is generally suitable for individuals of all ages, and there is no strict age restriction. It is particularly beneficial for seniors, individuals with mobility issues, and those seeking a gentle form of exercise. The key is to adapt the practice to individual needs and abilities.

Considerations:

- Tailored to All Ages: Chair yoga can be tailored to meet the needs of various age groups, from seniors to younger individuals with specific health concerns.

- Individual Adaptations: Instructors can provide modifications to accommodate different age groups and abilities.

- Mindful Practice: Regardless of age, participants should engage in chair yoga mindfully, respecting their bodies' limitations and finding a practice that suits their comfort level.

Additional Tips:

- Instructor Guidance: Seek guidance from a certified chair yoga instructor, especially if you're new to the practice or have specific health considerations.

- Community Support: Consider practicing chair yoga in a group setting to foster a sense of community and mutual support.

- Consistency is Key: Regular, consistent practice yields more significant benefits. Aim for a sustainable routine that you can maintain over the long term.

Chair yoga is a versatile and adaptable practice that can be enjoyed by individuals of all ages and abilities. Consulting with healthcare professionals, practicing at a comfortable frequency, and adapting poses to individual needs are key elements for a safe and enjoyable chair yoga experience.

CHAPTER TWELVE

Chair Yoga for Specific Health Conditions

These sequences are general guidelines, and individuals with these conditions should consult with their healthcare professionals before starting any new exercise program. A certified yoga instructor, preferably one with experience in therapeutic or chair yoga, can also provide personalized guidance and modifications.

A. **Chair Yoga for Arthritis:**

Objective: Improve joint mobility, reduce stiffness, and enhance overall well-being.

1. **Seated Neck Stretches:**

 Gently tilt the head from side to side, and forward and backward to release tension in the neck.

2. **Wrist and Hand Exercises:**

Rotate wrists and perform gentle hand stretches to alleviate stiffness.

3. **Seated Cat-Cow Stretch:**

Move through seated cat-cow stretches to promote flexibility in the spine and relieve tension in the back.

4. **Gentle Leg Lifts**:

Lift and lower each leg individually to engage the muscles around the hips and knees.

5. **Deep Breathing Exercise:**

Practice deep belly breathing to promote relaxation and reduce stress.

6. **Guided Relaxation:**

Finish with a guided relaxation to further release tension and promote a sense of calm.

B. Chair Yoga for Lower Back Pain

Objective: Strengthen and stretch the lower back muscles, and improve overall spinal health.

1. **Seated Forward Bend:**

Hinge at the hips and reach towards the toes, keeping the back straight to stretch the lower back.

2. **Seated Twist:**

Twist to each side, holding onto the back of the chair for support, to release tension in the lower back.

3. **Pelvic Tilts:**

Sit on the edge of the chair and gently tilt the pelvis forward and backward to engage the core and stretch the lower back.

4. **Seated Cat-Cow Stretch:**

Perform seated cat-cow stretches to enhance flexibility in the spine.

5. **Deep Breathing and Relaxation:**

Practice deep breathing exercises to promote relaxation, and finish with a guided relaxation.

C. **Chair Yoga for Stress and Anxiety**

Objective: Promote relaxation, reduce stress, and cultivate a sense of calm.

1. **Deep Breathing Exercises:**

Practice mindful breathing, focusing on slow inhalations and exhalations.

2. **Guided Relaxation:**

Sit comfortably and guide participants through a relaxation script, encouraging them to release tension from head to toe.

3. **Meditation in a Chair:**

Introduce a short meditation session, focusing on calming the mind and being present in the moment.

4. **Gentle Stretches:**

Incorporate gentle stretches for the neck, shoulders, and back to release physical tension.

5. **Chair Yoga Poses for Relaxation:**

Include poses like seated mountain pose and supported forward bend to create a calming atmosphere.

End the session with positive affirmations and encouragement to carry the sense of calm into daily life.

D. **Chair Yoga for Osteoporosis**

Objective: Promote bone health, increase strength, and improve posture.

1. **Seated Mountain Pose:**

Emphasize the importance of sitting tall with proper alignment to support the spine.

2. **Seated Leg Lifts**:

Lift and lower each leg individually to engage the muscles around the hips and strengthen the legs.

3. **Chair Squats:**

Perform chair squats with a focus on maintaining good posture to strengthen the lower body.

4. **Seated Twist with Back Support:**

Add back support for seated twists to enhance spinal mobility without straining the back.

5. Balancing on One Leg with Chair Support:

Stand behind the chair and practice balancing on one leg with the support of the chair to improve balance.

6. Deep Breathing and Relaxation:

Include deep breathing exercises for relaxation, and finish with a guided relaxation.

5. Chair Yoga for Diabetes

Objective: Promote circulation, improve flexibility, and reduce stress.

1. Seated Knee Lifts:

Lift and lower each knee individually to engage the muscles and promote circulation.

2. Ankle and Toe Flexibility:

Rotate ankles and flex toes to enhance circulation in the lower extremities

3. Chair Squats:

Perform controlled chair squats to engage leg muscles and improve overall circulation.

4. Seated Forward Bend:

Hinge at the hips for a seated forward bend to stretch the back and improve flexibility.

5. Deep Breathing and Relaxation:

Practice deep belly breathing to support relaxation and stress reduction.

6. Guided Relaxation:

Finish with a guided relaxation to promote overall well-being and reduce stress.

Notes:

- *Individual Modifications:* Participants should modify poses based on their comfort level and health status.

- *Regular Consultation:* Regularly consult with healthcare professionals to ensure that the chair yoga practice aligns with individual health conditions.

- *Consistent Practice*: Consistency is key. Encourage participants to maintain a regular chair yoga practice for long-term benefits.

Remember, these chair yoga sequences are general guidelines, and modifications should be made based on individual needs and abilities. Always prioritize safety, and participants with specific health concerns should consult with their healthcare professionals before starting any new exercise program. A certified chair yoga instructor can provide additional guidance and support.

"The pose begins when you want to leave it."
- B.K.S. Iyengar

CHAPTER THIRTEEN

Chair Yoga Warm up Movements

Warming up is crucial before engaging in any physical activity, including chair yoga. A good warm-up prepares the body for movement, increases blood flow to the muscles, and helps prevent injuries. Here are some chair yoga warm-up movements that you can incorporate into your routine:

1. Seated Neck Stretches:

- Sit with a straight spine.

- Inhale, lengthen the neck, and exhale, gently tilt the head to one side.

- Hold for a few breaths, feeling the stretch along the side of the neck.

- Repeat on the other side.

2. Seated Shoulder Rolls:

- Sit comfortably with hands on knees.

- Inhale, lift the shoulders up towards the ears.

- Exhale, roll the shoulders back and down.

- Repeat for 1-2 minutes to release tension.

3. Seated Side-to-Side Twists:

- Inhale, lengthen the spine.

- Exhale, twist gently to one side, holding onto the back of the chair for support.

- Inhale back to center and repeat on the other side.

4. Seated Arm Circles:

- Extend arms to the sides at shoulder height.

- Make small circles with the arms in a clockwise direction for 30 seconds.

- Reverse the direction for another 30 seconds.

5. Seated Hip Circles:

- Sit forward on the chair.

- Inhale, lift one knee towards the chest.

- Exhale, rotate the knee in a circular motion.

- Repeat for 30 seconds and switch to the other leg.

6. **Seated Knee Hugs:**

- Sit with a straight spine.

- Inhale, lift one knee towards the chest, hugging it with both hands.

- Exhale, lower the leg and switch to the other side.

7. **Seated Ankle Rolls:**

- Lift one foot off the ground and rotate the ankle in both directions.

- Switch to the other foot.

8. **Seated Forward and Backward Bends:**

- Inhale, lengthen the spine.

- Exhale, hinge at the hips and lean forward slightly.

- Inhale, sit back up, arching the spine.

- Repeat for 1-2 minutes.

9. **Seated Butterfly Stretch:**

- Bring the soles of the feet together, allowing the knees to drop to the sides.

- Hold the feet and gently press the knees towards the floor.

10. **Seated Marching:**

- Sit with feet flat on the ground.

- Inhale, lift one knee towards the chest.

- Exhale, lower the foot and lift the other knee.

- Continue alternating for 1-2 minutes.

Tips for Warm-Up Movements:

- Mindful Breathing: Encourage participants to synchronize movements with deep, slow breaths.

- Gentle Movements: Emphasize the importance of gentle and controlled movements to avoid strain.

- Full Range of Motion: Encourage participants to explore the full range of motion within their comfort zone.

- Individual Adaptations: Remind participants to modify movements based on their unique needs and abilities.

Incorporate these warm-up movements into your chair yoga sessions to ensure a safe and effective practice for participants.

11. **Seated Chest Opener:**

   - Sit with a straight spine.

   - Clasp hands behind your back, arms straight.

   - Inhale, lift the chest, and open the shoulders by squeezing the shoulder blades together.

   - Hold for a few breaths, feeling a stretch across the chest.

12. **Seated Side Leg Stretch:**

   - Sit with legs extended wide.

   - Inhale, lengthen the spine.

   - Exhale, reach towards one foot, feeling a stretch along the side of the body.

   - Hold for a few breaths and switch sides.

13. **Seated Torso Twist:**

   - Sit with a straight spine.

   - Inhale, raise both arms overhead.

   - Exhale, twist to one side, bringing one hand to the opposite knee and the other hand to the back of the chair.

   - Inhale back to center and repeat on the other side.

14. **Seated Wrist and Hand Exercises:**

   - Extend arms forward, flex and extend the wrists.

- Rotate the wrists clockwise and then counterclockwise.

- Open and close the fingers, moving each finger individually.

15. Seated Leg Swings:

- Sit at the edge of the chair.

- Swing one leg forward and backward, allowing it to gently lift off the floor.

- Switch to the other leg.

- Continue for 1-2 minutes.

16. Seated High Knees:

- Sit with a straight spine.

- Lift one knee towards the chest and hold for a moment.

- Lower and switch to the other knee.

- Continue alternating for 1-2 minutes.

17. **Seated Back Stretch:**

- Sit with a straight spine.

- Interlace fingers and extend arms forward, rounding the back.

- Hold for a few breaths, feeling a stretch between the shoulder blades.

18. **Seated Arm Stretch:**

- Sit with a straight spine.

- Bring one arm across the chest, using the opposite hand to gently press the arm towards the chest.

- Hold for a few breaths and switch sides.

19. **Seated Leg Cross Stretch:**

- Cross one leg over the other and hug the knee towards the chest.

- Hold for a few breaths, feeling a stretch in the outer hip.

- Switch to the other leg.

20. **Seated Gentle Bounce:**

   - Sit with feet flat on the ground.

   - Lift and drop the heels rhythmically, creating a gentle bouncing motion.

   - Continue for 1-2 minutes to promote circulation.

Tips for Incorporating Warm-Up Movements
- Fluid Transitions: Encourage participants to move smoothly from one warm-up movement to the next.

- Body Awareness: Emphasize the importance of paying attention to how the body feels during the warm-up.

- Gradual Intensity: Start with gentler movements and gradually progress to more dynamic ones as the warm-up continues.

- Personalization: Remind participants to adapt movements based on their comfort level and any existing physical conditions.

Incorporating these warm-up movements into your chair yoga sessions will enhance the overall experience for participants, ensuring a safe and enjoyable practice. Warm-ups prepare the body and mind for the upcoming yoga session, setting the stage for a positive and beneficial experience.

"It's never too late, and you're never too old to become better." - Bikram Choudhury

CHAPTER FOURTEEN
Nutritional Diet for Chair Yoga for seniors

Well-balanced and nutritious diet is essential for seniors over 60, including those engaging in chair yoga. Proper nutrition supports overall health, provides energy, and aids in recovery. Here are some key nutritional considerations for seniors practicing chair yoga:

1. Hydration:

Importance: Staying hydrated is crucial for overall health, especially as aging adults may be more prone to dehydration.

Recommendations: Aim for at least 8 glasses (64 ounces) of water per day. Adjust based on individual needs, considering factors like climate and activity levels.

2. Balanced Diet:

Importance: Ensure a well-rounded diet to provide essential nutrients for overall health and vitality.

Recommendations: Include a variety of fruits and vegetables for vitamins, minerals, and antioxidants. Incorporate whole grains for fiber and sustained energy. Include lean proteins like poultry, fish, beans, and tofu for muscle maintenance and repair.

3. **Protein Intake:**

Importance: Adequate protein is essential for maintaining muscle mass and supporting recovery from physical activity.

Recommendations: Include protein-rich foods in each meal, such as eggs, dairy, lean meats, legumes, and nuts.

4. Calcium and Vitamin D:

Importance: Essential for bone health, especially important for seniors to prevent osteoporosis.

Recommendations: Include dairy products, leafy green vegetables, and fortified foods for calcium. Spend time in sunlight for natural vitamin D or consider a supplement if needed.

5. **Omega-3 Fatty Acids:**

Importance: Supportive of heart health, joint function, and cognitive well-being.

Recommendations: Include fatty fish (salmon, mackerel) or fish oil supplements. Incorporate walnuts, flaxseeds, and chia seeds into the diet.

6. Fiber:

Importance: Aids in digestion, supports heart health, and helps maintain a healthy weight.

Recommendations: Include whole grains, fruits, vegetables, and legumes in the diet.

7. Antioxidant-Rich Foods:

Importance: Protect cells from oxidative stress and support overall health.

Recommendations: Include colorful fruits and vegetables such as berries, spinach, kale, and bell peppers.

8. Limit Processed Foods and Added Sugars:

Importance: Reducing the intake of processed foods and added sugars supports overall health and weight management.

Recommendations: Opt for whole, minimally processed foods and limit sugary snacks and beverages.

9. Meal Timing:

Importance: Eating regular, balanced meals supports stable energy levels and overall well-being.

Recommendations: Aim for three balanced meals with healthy snacks if needed, spaced throughout the day.

10. Consider Individual Needs:

Importance: Individual nutritional needs may vary based on health conditions, medications, and personal preferences.

Recommendations: Consult with a healthcare professional or a registered dietitian for personalized guidance.

Additional Tips:

Pre-Exercise Nutrition: Consume a light, balanced meal or snack about 1-2 hours before chair yoga to provide energy.

Post-Exercise Nutrition: Include a source of protein after chair yoga to support muscle recovery. This could be a protein-rich snack or part of a meal.

Sample Day of Nutritious Meals

Breakfast:

- Oatmeal with berries and a sprinkle of nuts.

- Greek yogurt with sliced banana.

- Herbal tea or water.

Lunch:

- Grilled chicken or tofu salad with mixed greens, tomatoes, cucumbers, and olive oil dressing.

- Quinoa or whole-grain roll on the side.

- Water or herbal tea.

Snack:

- Handful of mixed nuts and seeds.

- Apple slices with a small amount of peanut butter.

- Water or herbal tea.

Dinner:

- Baked salmon or a vegetarian stir-fry with tofu and colorful vegetables.

- Brown rice or sweet potato on the side.

- Steamed broccoli or green beans.

- Water or herbal tea.

Note: Adjust portion sizes based on individual needs and preferences.

Remember, nutrition is a highly individualized aspect of health. It's advisable for seniors to consult with a healthcare professional or a registered dietitian for personalized advice based on their specific health conditions and dietary requirements.

Yoga is the journey of the self, through the self, to the self." - The Bhagavad Gita

CHAPTER FIFTEEN
Chair Cardio Exercises for Weight Loss

Chair cardio exercises can be an effective and accessible way for individuals with mobility challenges or those who prefer seated workouts to engage in cardiovascular activity. These exercises can contribute to weight loss when combined with a healthy diet and overall active lifestyle. Here's a chair cardio workout that focuses on raising the heart rate, improving circulation, and burning calories:

Warm-Up (2-3 minutes)
1. Seated March:

  - Sit tall with feet flat on the floor.

  - Lift one knee and then the other in a marching motion.

  - Engage the core and swing the arms gently.

2. Arm Circles:

  - Extend arms to the sides.

- Make small circles in a clockwise direction, then switch to counterclockwise.

3. Seated Toe Taps:

   - Sit with a straight spine.

   - Tap one foot on the floor and then the other, alternating in a rhythmic motion.

Cardio Exercises (20-30 minutes)
1. Seated Jumping Jacks:

   - Lift arms overhead and open the legs wide simultaneously.

   - Lower arms and bring legs together.

   - Repeat in a jumping jack motion while seated.

2. Seated High Knees:

   - Sit tall and lift one knee towards the chest.

   - Alternate quickly between legs, creating a high-knee motion while engaging the core.

3. Seated Side Leg Lifts:

- Sit with feet together.

- Lift one leg to the side, engaging the outer thigh.

- Lower and repeat on the other side.

4. Seated Cross Punches:

- Sit tall and extend one arm across the body while twisting the torso.

- Alternate sides, engaging the core with each punch.

5. Seated Butt Kicks:

- Sit tall and kick one heel towards the glutes.

- Alternate legs in a quick-paced motion.

6. Seated Knee Extensions:

- Sit with a straight spine and extend one leg at a time, lifting it off the floor.

- Alternate between legs in a continuous motion.

1. **Seated Torso Twist:**

   - Sit tall and twist gently to one side, holding onto the back of the chair for support.

   - Repeat on the other side.

2. **Deep Breathing:**

   - Inhale deeply through the nose, expanding the belly.

   - Exhale slowly through pursed lips, focusing on calming the breath.

3. **Shoulder Rolls:**

   - Inhale, lift the shoulders towards the ears.

   - Exhale, roll them back and down in a smooth motion.

4. **Seated Forward Bend:**

- Inhale, lengthen the spine.

- Exhale, hinge at the hips, reaching towards the toes for a gentle stretch.

Tips for Chair Cardio

1. **Maintain Good Posture**: Sit tall with shoulders relaxed and spine straight throughout the workout.

2. **Engage Core Muscles**: Tighten the abdominal muscles to support the spine and enhance the effectiveness of the exercises.

3. **Modify Intensity:** Adjust the speed and range of motion based on individual fitness levels and comfort.

4. **Consistency is Key**: Aim for at least 20-30 minutes of chair cardio most days of the week for optimal results.

5. **Stay Hydrated:** Drink water before, during, and after the workout to stay hydrated.

6. **Listen to Your Body**: If any exercise causes discomfort or pain, modify or skip that movement.

7. **Combine with a Balanced Diet:** Pair chair cardio with a healthy, well-balanced diet to support weight loss goals.

Always consult with a healthcare professional before starting a new exercise routine, especially if you have any existing health conditions. Adjust the duration and intensity of the workout to match individual fitness levels and gradually increase the challenge as endurance improves.

"Yoga is invigoration in relaxation. Freedom in routine. Confidence through self-control. Energy within and energy without." - Ymber Delecto

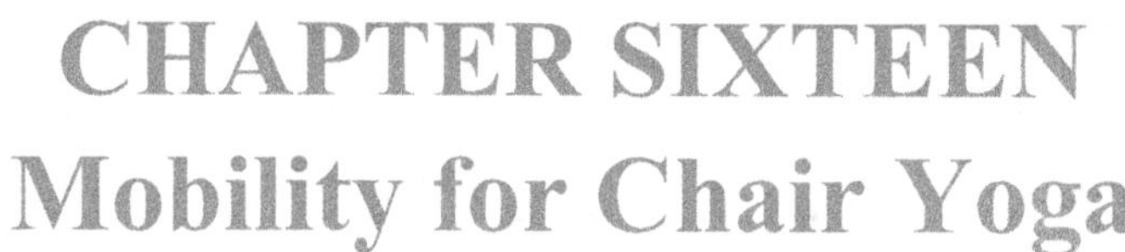

CHAPTER SIXTEEN
Mobility for Chair Yoga

Enhancing mobility is a key focus in chair yoga, especially for seniors or individuals with limited mobility. Chair yoga offers a gentle and accessible way to improve flexibility, joint range of motion, and overall mobility. Here's a guide on enhancing mobility through chair yoga:

1. Gentle Warm-Up Movements:

- Start with seated neck stretches, shoulder rolls, and wrist rotations to gently warm up the upper body.

- Include seated ankle rolls, knee lifts, and hip circles to warm up the lower body.

2. Focus on Breath Awareness:

- Encourage participants to sync their movements with deep, intentional breaths.

- Deep breathing promotes relaxation and can enhance the effectiveness of mobility exercises.

3. **Seated Cat-Cow Stretch:**

- Inhale, arch the back, and lift the chest (Cow).

- Exhale, round the back and bring the chin to the chest (Cat).

- Repeat in a flowing motion to mobilize the spine.

4. **Seated Forward Bend:**

- Inhale, lengthen the spine.

- Exhale, hinge at the hips, reaching towards the toes to stretch the back and hamstrings.

5. **Seated Side Stretch:**

- Inhale, reach one arm overhead.

- Exhale, lean to the side, feeling a stretch along the torso.

- Repeat on the other side to improve lateral mobility.

6. **Seated Twist:**

- Inhale, lengthen the spine.

- Exhale, twist to one side, using the back of the chair for support.

- Inhale back to center and repeat on the other side to enhance spinal rotation.

7. **Neck Stretches:**

- Gently tilt the head from side to side and forward and backward to increase neck mobility.

- Rotate the head clockwise and counterclockwise to address different ranges of motion.

8. **Chair Sun Salutation:**

Flow through a modified sun salutation while seated, incorporating arm raises, forward bends, and twists to enhance overall mobility.

9. **Seated Butterfly Stretch:**

Bring the soles of the feet together, holding onto the ankles. Gently press the knees towards the floor to stretch the inner thighs and hips.

10. Modified Tree Pose:

- Lift one foot and place the sole against the inner thigh or calf of the opposite leg.

- Hold onto the back of the chair for support to improve balance and hip mobility.

11. Seated Leg Lifts:

Sit tall and lift one leg at a time, engaging the quadriceps and improving hip flexibility.

12. Adapt Poses for Comfort:

Encourage participants to use props like cushions or blocks to modify poses for comfort and support.

13. **Progressive Movement Patterns:**

Gradually introduce more complex movements, combining gentle stretches with controlled joint movements to enhance overall mobility.

14. **Focus on Alignment:**

Emphasize proper alignment to prevent strain and ensure the targeted muscle groups are engaged during each movement.

15. **Mindful Movements:**

Encourage participants to perform each movement mindfully, paying attention to how their body responds and adapting accordingly.

16. **Consistency is Key:**

Consistent practice is crucial for improving mobility. Encourage participants to integrate chair yoga into their routine several times a week.

17. **Provide Individual Support:**

Offer individualized guidance and modifications based on each participant's unique mobility challenges and goals.

18. **Cool Down and Relaxation:**

Finish the session with gentle stretches and relaxation poses to ease tension and promote a sense of calm.

19. **Consult with a Professional:**

For individuals with specific mobility concerns or health conditions, recommend consulting with a healthcare professional or physical therapist for personalized guidance.

20. **Celebrate Progress:**

Encourage participants to celebrate small victories and improvements in mobility, fostering a positive mindset towards their practice.

By incorporating these principles into chair yoga sessions, you can create a supportive and effective environment for enhancing mobility. Regular practice will contribute to improved flexibility, joint range of motion, and overall well-being.

Thanks for your purchase, hope you enjoyed reading.

Could you please take a few seconds to leave a positive feedback on this book?

It will help reach out to more people especially seniors above 60 and help them steady and younger.

Stay
Healthy
Always!!!

www.ingramcontent.com/pod-product-compliance
Lightning Source LLC
Chambersburg PA
CBHW080927260726
48661CB00010B/3824